THE LIVER CIRRHOSIS DIET COOKBOOK 2024

Easy, Delicious and Nutritious Healing Recipes For Improving Liver Health & Ensuring Overall Wellbeing

21 day meal plan

MILDRED BELS

TABLE OF CONTENTS

One

Overview of Nutrition and Liver Health

One of the most important organs in the human body is the liver, which performs a wide range of necessary tasks that keep us healthy. If liver cirrhosis is not adequately treated, it might result in liver failure due to the condition's increasing scarring of the liver. Here, we will cover the fundamentals of liver health, the role that diet plays in supporting liver function, and key advice for sticking to a diet that is good for the liver.

Liver cirrhosis is a late stage of liver fibrosis, or scarring, brought on by a variety of liver illnesses and disorders, including prolonged alcoholism and hepatitis. The liver's ability to operate normally is hampered when the scarring intensifies. Liver failure and liver cancer are just two of the many consequences that can result from cirrhosis.

Liver cirrhosis can cause a variety of symptoms, such as weakness, fatigue, appetite loss, easy bruising, and jaundice (yellowing of the skin and eyes). It's vital to remember that liver cirrhosis may not exhibit any symptoms in its early stages, making routine screenings and examinations essential for early identification and treatment.

✓ Nutrition's Significance for Liver Health

Maintaining liver health is mostly dependent on eating a well-balanced diet, particularly for those who have liver cirrhosis. In addition to supporting general liver function, proper nutrition can help manage symptoms and lower the risk of problems. The following are some important food factors for liver health:

1.   **Restricting   Sodium   Intake:**
Consuming too much sodium can cause fluid retention, which can be dangerous for people who have liver cirrhosis. Reducing sodium consumption can assist in controlling fluid accumulation and lower the chance of consequences such as ascites (abdominal fluid buildup).

2. **Moderating Protein Intake:** Protein is necessary to sustain general health and muscular mass. However, as too much protein can strain the liver, those with liver cirrhosis may need to restrict their protein intake. It is advised to consume high-quality

protein sources such fish, poultry, eggs, lean meats, and plant-based proteins.

3. **Selecting Healthful Fats:** Nuts, seeds, avocados, and olive oil are good sources of healthy fats that promote general wellbeing and liver health. Because of their high antioxidant and anti-inflammatory content, these fats may help lessen liver damage and inflammation.

4. **Reducing Alcohol Consumption:** People with liver cirrhosis should avoid or use alcohol in moderation as it is a key cause of liver damage. When

cirrhosis reaches an advanced stage, alcohol should be completely avoided as even little amounts can be detrimental to the liver.

5. **Consuming a Range of Fruits and Vegetables:** Fruits and vegetables are a great source of antioxidants, vitamins, and minerals that are beneficial to liver function. They also include fiber, which can lessen the likelihood of constipation, a major problem among people with liver cirrhosis, and aid in better digestion.

Eating a balanced diet is not the only thing necessary to maintain a healthy liver. Here are a few more suggestions to help maintain liver health:

1. **Maintain Proper Hydration:** Liver health depends on proper hydration. Water facilitates digestion and aids in the removal of toxins from the body.

2. **Engage in Regular Exercise:** Exercise on a regular basis can help lower liver fat, increase insulin sensitivity, and enhance general health. On most days of the week, try

to get in at least 30 minutes of moderate activity.

3. **Steer clear of fad diets**: Although they frequently lack vital nutrients and promote rapid weight reduction, which can strain the liver, fad diets can be detrimental to liver health.

4. **Get Regular Check-ups**: It's critical to visit your doctor on a regular basis to monitor the condition of your liver and identify any possible problems early on.

5. **Quit Smoking**: Smoking raises the risk of liver cancer and exacerbates

liver damage. Giving up smoking can help you feel better overall and protect your liver.

People with liver cirrhosis can enhance their quality of life and lower their risk of problems by learning the fundamentals of liver health, the role that nutrition plays in supporting liver function, and how to maintain a good liver diet.

Two

Breakfast Recipes

✓ Avocado Toast with Poached Eggs

Ingredients:

- One ripe avocado

- Two pieces of whole grain bread

- Two sizable eggs

- Topping suggestions: cherry tomatoes, red pepper flakes, and microgreens.

- Season with salt and pepper to suit.

Instructions:

1. Toast the slices of whole grain bread till golden brown.

2. Bring a pot of water to a simmer and poach the eggs while the bread is toasting. After gently cracking each egg into a small bowl, place them in the water that is simmering. Cook until the yolk is soft, 3 to 4 minutes.

3. Use a fork to mash the ripe avocado in a bowl until it's smooth while the eggs are poaching. To taste, add salt and pepper for seasoning.

4. Evenly distribute the mashed avocado over the slices of toasted bread.

5. Using a slotted spoon, carefully take the cooked eggs from the water and arrange them atop the avocado toast.

6. Add optional garnishes like microgreens, cherry tomatoes, or red pepper flakes.

7. Serve right away.

Two servings

Ten minutes to cook

Nutritional Value: 320 calories per serving

14g of protein

- 26g of carbohydrates

- 20g of fat

- 9g of fiber

✓ *Almonds and Berries with Oatmeal*

Ingredients:

- One cup water or your preferred milk

- Half a cup rolled oats

- A half cup of mixed berries, including raspberries, blueberries, and strawberries

- One tablespoon of almonds, sliced

- Optional garnishes: chia seeds, honey, and cinnamon

Instructions:

1. Bring the milk or water to a boil in a small saucepan.

2. Turn down the heat and stir in the rolled oats. Cook, stirring periodically, until the oats become thick and creamy, about 5 to 7 minutes.

3. Take the oats off of the stove and put it in a bowl.

4. Sprinkle sliced almonds and mixed berries over the oatmeal.

5. You can optionally drizzle honey or add cinnamon or chia seeds, if you'd like.

6. Present warm.

One serving

Ten minutes to cook

Nutritional Value:

- 300 calories per serving

- 10g of protein

- 45g of carbohydrates

- 9g of fat

- 8g of fiber

✓ *Omelet with spinach and mushrooms*

Ingredients:

- Two sizable eggs

- 1/2 cup sliced mushrooms

- 1 cup chopped fresh spinach

- 1/4 cup of feta or cheddar cheese, shredded

- To taste, add salt and pepper. Use one teaspoon of olive oil.

Instructions:

1. Beat the eggs with the salt and pepper in a small bowl until thoroughly mixed.

2. In a nonstick skillet, warm the olive oil over medium heat.

3. Add the sliced mushrooms and chopped spinach to the skillet. Cook for two to three minutes, or until the mushrooms are soft and the spinach has wilted.

4. To achieve equitable distribution, pour the beaten eggs over the spinach

and mushrooms while turning the skillet.

5. Fry the omelet for two to three minutes, or until the sides begin to firm.

6. Top half of the omelette with the shredded cheese.

7. Fold the remaining omelette over the cheese with a spatula.

8. Cook for a further one to two minutes, or until the eggs are fully cooked and the cheese has melted.

9. Transfer the omelet to a platter and enjoy it warm.

One serving

Ten minutes to cook

Nutritional Value: 280 calories per serving

20g of protein

- 6g of carbohydrates

- 20g of fat

- 2g of fiber

✓ *Parfait of Greek Yogurt with Granola and Honey*

Ingredients:

- One cup of Greek yogurt

- 1/4 cup of granola

- 1/4 cup mixed berries (strawberries, blueberries, raspberries)

- 1 tablespoon honey

Instructions:

1. Arrange the Greek yogurt, granola, and mixed berries in a glass or bowl.

2. Pour honey over the top.

3. Continue layering until all of the ingredients have been utilized. Finish by drizzling honey over the top.

4. Present right away.

Servings: 1; 5-minute prep

Nutritional Value:

- 300 calories per serving

20g of protein

- 35g of carbohydrates

- 10g of fat

- 4g of fiber

Ingredients:

- One cup of whole wheat flour

- One tablespoon of powdered sugar

- One tablespoon maple syrup or honey

- One cup any type of milk

- One big egg

- One tsp of vanilla extract

- Butter or cooking spray to coat the pan

- Fresh fruit (such as cut berries or bananas) to garnish

Instructions:

1. Combine the baking powder and whole wheat flour in a large basin.

2. In another dish, thoroughly whisk together the milk, egg, vanilla extract, and honey/maple syrup.

3. Add the wet mixture to the dry mixture and whisk just until blended. It's alright to have some lumps; don't overmix.

4. Apply a thin layer of cooking spray or butter to a non-stick skillet or griddle before heating it to medium heat.

5. For each pancake, pour 1/4 cup of batter into the skillet.

6. Cook for two to three minutes, or until bubbles appear on the pancake's surface and the edges start to firm.

7. After flipping the pancakes, heat for a further one to two minutes, or until they are cooked through and golden brown.

8. Continue with the leftover batter.

9. If desired, top the pancakes with fresh fruit and a sprinkle of maple syrup or honey.

Serves two to three (makes roughly six pancakes)

15 minutes is the cooking time.

Value for nutrition (per serving, omitting toppings):

- 220 calories

- 9g of protein

- 35g of carbohydrates

- 5g of fat

- 4g of fiber

✓ *Fantastic Breakfast Bowl of Quinoa with Nuts and Seeds*

Ingredients:

- 1/4 cup Greek yogurt

- 1/2 cup cooked quinoa

- One tablespoon of maple syrup or honey

- 1/4 cup of assorted nuts and seeds, including sunflower, walnut, almond, and pumpkin seeds

- One-fourth cup assorted berries, including raspberries, blueberries, and strawberries

- Optional garnishes include cinnamon, chopped coconut, and banana slices.

Instructions:

1. Put the cooked quinoa, Greek yogurt, and maple syrup or honey in a bowl.

2. Ensure that the quinoa is thoroughly mixed and coated.

3. Add mixed nuts and seeds, mixed berries, and any additional optional toppings to the quinoa mixture.

4. Present right away.

Servings: 1; 5-minute prep

Nutritional Value: 350 calories per serving

- 15g of protein

- 45g of carbohydrates

- 15g of fat

- 6g of fiber

✓ *Cream cheese and smoked salmon bagel*

Ingredients:

- Two tablespoons cream cheese

- One whole grain or everything bagel, sliced and toasted

- Two ounces of salmon smoked

- One tablespoon of capers

- 1/4 thinly sliced red onion

- Fresh dill for garnish

Instructions:

1. Evenly spread cream cheese over both toasted bagel halves.

2. Place thinly sliced red onion, capers, and smoked salmon on top of one half of the bagel.

3. Add fresh dill as a garnish.

4. To create a sandwich, place the second half of the bagel on top.

5. Present right away.

Servings: 1; 5-minute prep

Nutritional Value: 380 calories per serving

20g of protein

- 45g of carbohydrates

- 15g of fat

- 4g of fiber

Ingredients:

- 1/4 cup walnuts

- 1 ripe banana, peeled and sliced

- Half a cup of Greek yogurt

- 1/2 cup your preferred milk

- 1 tablespoon maple syrup or honey

- One-fourth teaspoon of cinnamon

- Ice cubes, if desired

Instructions:

1. Place the banana slices, walnuts, Greek yogurt, milk, cinnamon, honey, or maple syrup in a blender.

2. Blend until creamy and smooth. To make the smoothie colder, feel free to add ice cubes.

3. Immediately serve after pouring into a glass.

Servings: 1; 5-minute prep

Nutritional Value: 380 calories per serving

- 15g of protein

- 45g of carbohydrates

- 15g of fat

- 5g of fiber

✓ *Breakfast Burrito with Veggies*

Ingredients:

- One tortilla, either spinach or whole wheat

- 2 big scrambled eggs

- 1/4 cup rinsed and drained black beans

- 1/4 cup diced tomatoes

- 1/4 cup diced bell peppers

- 2 tablespoons diced red onion

- 1/4 cup shredded cheese (like Monterey Jack or cheddar)

- Avocado and salsa to serve (optional)

Instructions:

1. In a skillet over medium heat, cook the tortilla until it's fully heated.

2. Evenly distribute the scrambled eggs onto the tortilla.

3. Add shredded cheese, chopped tomatoes, diced red onion, diced bell peppers, and black beans on top.

4. To construct a burrito, fold in the tortilla's sides and roll it tightly.

5. If preferred, top with avocado and salsa and serve.

Servings: 1; 10-minute prep

Nutritional Value: 380 calories per serving

20g of protein

- 35g of carbohydrates

- 18g of fat

- 8g of fiber

✓ *Mango-Chia Seed Pudding*

Ingredients:

- One-fourth cup chia seeds

- One cup of choice of milk

- One ripe mango, diced

- One tablespoon honey or maple syrup

- Half a teaspoon vanilla extract

Instructions:

1. Combine the milk, vanilla extract, honey (or maple syrup), and chia seeds in a bowl.

2. Continue to cover and chill the mixture for at least two hours, or overnight, until it thickens and takes on the consistency of pudding.

3. Give the chia seed pudding a stir to make sure it's smooth and well combined.

4. Ladle the pudding made with chia seeds into glasses or serving dishes.

5. Add diced mango on top.

6. Present cold.

Two servings

Prepare Time: five minutes, including cooling off

Value of Nutrition (per serving):

- 220 calories

- 5g of protein

- 35g of carbohydrates

- 8g of fat

- 10g of fiber

These breakfast recipes provide you a range of tasty and nourishing options to make sure your day gets off to a good start! Enjoy playing around with these tastes and components.

Three

Lunch Recipes

✓ Mixed greens with Grilled Chicken Salad

Ingredients:

- One skinless and boneless chicken breast

- Four cups of mixed greens (such as kale, spinach, and arugula)

- Salt and pepper to taste

- 1/4 cup sliced cucumber

- 1/2 cup chopped cherry tomatoes

- 1/4 cup diced bell peppers

- Two teaspoons of crumbled feta cheese

– Two tsp balsamic vinaigrette

Instructions:

1. Turn the heat up to medium-high on a grill or grill pan.

2. Use salt and pepper to season the chicken breast.

3. Grill the chicken breast for 6 to 8 minutes on each side, or until it is well cooked and the middle is no longer pink.

4. Take the chicken off the grill, let it a few minutes to rest, and then thinly slice it.

5. Combine the bell peppers, cucumber, cherry tomatoes, and grilled chicken slices in a big bowl together with the mixed greens.

6. Coat evenly with balsamic vinaigrette by tossing.

7. Top with feta cheese crumbles.

8. Present right away.

One serving

Ten minutes for preparation

Cooking Period: 15 minutes

Value of Nutrition (per serving):

- 350 calories

- 30g of protein

- 15g of carbohydrates

- 18g of fat

- 5g of fiber

✓ *Lentil Soup with Tomatoes and Spinach*

Ingredients:

- One cup of rinsed and drained dried green lentils

- 4 cups vegetable broth

- 1 chopped onion

- 2 minced garlic cloves

- One chopped carrot

- One sliced celery stalk

- One 14-oz can of chopped tomatoes

- One teaspoon dried thyme

- Two cups fresh spinach

- Toppings of salt and pepper

Instructions:

1. Place the vegetable broth and dried lentils in a big pot.

2. Once the lentils are soft, reduce the heat to low and simmer for 20 to 25 minutes after bringing to a boil.

3. In a different skillet, soften the minced garlic and chopped onion with olive oil.

4. Add the onion and garlic that have been sautéed to the lentil pot.

5. Add the dried thyme, chopped tomatoes (with their liquids), diced carrot, diced celery, salt, and pepper.

6. Simmer the vegetables for ten to fifteen more minutes, or until they are soft.

7. Stir in the fresh spinach until it wilts.

8. Taste and adjust seasoning as necessary.

9. Present warm.

4 servings

Ten minutes for preparation

40 minutes for cooking

Value of Nutrition (per serving):

- 250 calories

- 15g of protein

- 40g of carbohydrates

- Fat: 2 g

- 15g of fiber

✓ *Avocado and Turkey Wrap*

Ingredients:

- One whole wheat tortilla

- 3 ounces of slices of deli turkey

- 1/4 sliced avocado

- 1/4 cup of chopped lettuce

- 1/4 cup of tomatoes, diced

- Two tablespoons of Greek yogurt spread or hummus

Instructions:

1. Place the whole-wheat tortilla flat on a spotlessly clean surface.

2. Evenly distribute hummus or Greek yogurt throughout the tortilla.

3. Arrange the chopped tomatoes, sliced avocado, shredded lettuce, and

deli turkey slices on top of the mixture.

4. Tightly roll the tortilla into a wrap.

5. If desired, cut the wrap in half diagonally.

6. Present right away.

Servings: 1; 5-minute prep

Nutritional Value:

- 300 calories per serving

- 20g of protein

- 30g of carbohydrates

- 12g of fat

- 8g of fiber

Ingredients:

- 1 can (15 oz) rinsed and drained black beans

- 1 cup cooked quinoa

- Half a cup of fresh, canned, or frozen corn kernels

- One-fourth cup of diced red and green bell peppers

- Two tablespoons of freshly chopped cilantro

- Two tablespoons of lime juice

- One tablespoon olive oil

- One teaspoon ground cumin

- Toppings: chopped tomatoes, shredded cheese, and avocado slices

- Salt and pepper to taste

Instructions:

1. Combine the cooked quinoa, black beans, corn kernels, diced green and red bell peppers, chopped fresh cilantro, and a big bowl.

2. Combine the lime juice, olive oil, ground cumin, salt, and pepper in a small bowl.

3. Drizzle the quinoa and black bean mixture with the dressing, tossing to coat evenly.

4. Taste and adjust spice as necessary.

5. Garnish with chopped tomatoes, shredded cheese, or avocado slices, and serve cold or room temperature.

4 servings

15 minutes for preparation

Cooking time for quinoa is 15 minutes.

Value of Nutrition (per serving):

- 250 calories

- 10g of protein

- 40g of carbohydrates

- 6g of fat

- 8g of fiber

✓ *Lettuce Wraps with Tuna Salad*

Ingredients:

- One 5-ounce tin of drained tuna

- Two tsp Greek yogurt

- One tablespoon of mayo

- One tablespoon Dijon mustard

- One-fourth cup chopped celery

- One-fourth cup diced red onion

- One tablespoon chopped parsley or fresh dill

- Four large lettuce leaves (such as butter lettuce or romaine)

- Salt and pepper to taste

Instructions:

1. Put the tuna that has been drained, Greek yogurt, mayonnaise, Dijon mustard, sliced onion, diced celery, and chopped parsley or fresh dill in a bowl.

2. Thoroughly stir until all items are combined.

3. To taste, add salt and pepper for seasoning.

4. Evenly divide the combination of tuna salad among the large lettuce leaves.

5. To make lettuce wraps, encircle the tuna salad mixture with the lettuce leaves.

6. Present right away.

Two servings

Ten minutes for preparation

Nutritional Value (2 lettuce wraps per serving):

- 150 calories

20g of protein

- 5g of carbohydrates

- 5g of fat

- 2g of fiber

✓ *Stir-fried Vegetables with Chickpeas*

Ingredients:

- 1 can (15 oz) rinsed and drained chickpeas

- 2 cups mixed veggies (carrots, broccoli, bell peppers, snap peas)

- 2 minced garlic cloves

- Two tablespoons of soy sauce (for a gluten-free option, use tamari).

- Prepared brown rice or quinoa for serving

- 1 tablespoon sesame oil

- 1 tablespoon rice vinegar

- 1 tablespoon honey or maple syrup

- 1 teaspoon grated ginger

- Optional toppings: sliced green onions, sesame seeds

Instructions:

1. In a large skillet or wok, heat the sesame oil over medium-high heat.

2. Sauté the grated ginger and minced garlic in the skillet for one minute, or until fragrant.

3. Add the mixed vegetables to the skillet and stir-fry until they are crisp-tender, about 3 to 4 minutes.

4. Stir-fry the chickpeas for a further two minutes after adding them to the skillet.

5. Combine the soy sauce, rice vinegar, and honey/maple syrup in a small bowl.

6. Drizzle the skillet's chickpea and veggie combination with the sauce.

7. Stir-fry the veggies and chickpeas for a further one to two minutes, or until the sauce thickens and covers them equally.

8. Turn off the heat and serve the stir-fry over quinoa or brown rice that has been cooked.

9. If preferred, garnish with sesame seeds and sliced green onions.

10. Present right away.

4 servings

Ten minutes for preparation

15 minutes is the cooking time.

Value for Nutrition (per serving, omitting quinoa and rice):

- 200 calories

- 8g of protein

- 25g of carbohydrates

- 8g of fat

- 6g of fiber

✓ *Salad Nicoise with Salmon*

Ingredients:

- 4 cups mixed salad greens

- 2 salmon fillets

- Salt & pepper to taste

- One cup of chopped cherry tomatoes

- Half a cup of cooled, cooked green beans

- 1/4 cup pitted Kalamata olives

- 2 sliced hard-boiled eggs

- Two teaspoons of capers.

- Serving wedges of lemon

- Optional attire: Maybe a balsamic or Dijon vinaigrette

Instructions:

1. Sprinkle salt and pepper on the salmon filets.

2. Place the skin-side down salmon filets into a heated skillet set over medium-high heat.

3. Until the salmon is cooked through and flake readily with a fork, grill it for 4–5 minutes on each side.

4. Take the salmon out of the skillet and give it a little time to cool.

5. Place the cooked green beans, cherry tomatoes, capers, sliced hard-boiled eggs, Kalamata olives, and mixed salad greens in a big bowl.

6. Add the cooked salmon to the salad by flaking it into chunks.

7. Garnish with optional dressing or present with wedges of lemon, if preferred.

8. Gently toss the salad to include all of the ingredients.

9. Present right away.

Two servings

15 minutes for preparation

Ten minutes to cook

Value of Nutrition (per serving):

- 350 calories

- 30g of protein

- 15g of carbohydrates

- 20g of fat

- 5g of fiber

✓ *Sweet Potato and Turkey Chili*

Ingredients:

- One tablespoon olive oil

- Diced onion

- Minced garlic cloves

- One pound of pounded turkey

- One fifteen-ounce can of rinsed and

drained black beans

- One 15-oz can of chopped tomatoes

- Two cups chicken broth

- One large sweet potato, peeled and chopped

- One tablespoon chile powder

- One teaspoon of ground cumin; salt and pepper to taste

- Optional toppings: sour cream, Greek yogurt, shredded cheese, or chopped green onions

Instructions:

1. In a large pot over medium heat, warm the olive oil.

2. Add the minced garlic and chopped onion to the pot and sauté for 3-4

minutes, or until the ingredients are tender.

3. Add the ground turkey to the saucepan and heat, breaking it up with a spoon, until it is browned.

4. Add the diced sweet potato, diced tomatoes, black beans, chicken broth, ground cumin, ground chili powder, and salt and pepper.

5. After bringing the chili to a boil, lower the heat to a simmer and cook the sweet potatoes for 20 to 25 minutes, or until they are soft.

6. Taste and adjust seasoning as necessary.

7. Garnish with shredded cheese, sliced green onions, Greek yogurt, or sour cream, if desired, and serve hot.

Six servings

Ten minutes for preparation

30 minutes for cooking

Value of Nutrition (per serving):

- 300 calories

25g of protein

- 30g of carbohydrates

- 10g of fat

- 8g of fiber

✓ *Grilled shrimp in a Greek salad*

Ingredients:

- 4 cups mixed salad greens

- 1 tablespoon olive oil

- 8 large shrimp, peeled and deveined

- Salt and pepper to taste

- Half a cucumber, cut

- 1/4 cup pitted Kalamata olives

- 1/2 cup chopped cherry tomatoes

- 1/4 cup crumbled feta cheese

- Lemon wedges to serve

- Dressing optional: Greek salad dressing

Instructions:

1. Turn the heat up to medium-high on a grill or grill pan.

2. Combine salt, pepper, and olive oil with the peeled and deveined shrimp.

3. Grill the shrimp until they are cooked through and pink, about two to three minutes per side.

4. Combine the mixed salad greens, cucumber slices, cherry tomatoes, feta cheese crumbles, and Kalamata olives in a big bowl.

5. Top the salad with the cooked shrimp.

6. Present the salad with optional Greek vinaigrette dressing on the side along with lemon wedges.

7. Gently toss the salad to include all of the ingredients.

8. Present right away.

Two servings

Ten minutes for preparation

Six minutes to cook

Value of Nutrition (per serving):

- 250 calories

- 20g of protein

- 15g of carbohydrates

- 12g of fat

- 4g of fiber

✓ **Sushi Rolls with Brown Rice and Vegetables**

Ingredients:

- Four sheets of nori seaweed

- 1/2 cucumber, thinly sliced

- 2 cups cooked brown rice

- Half of an avocado, cut

- 1/2 julienned carrot

- 1/4 julienned red bell pepper

- Four optional slices of tofu or crab sticks

- To serve, soy sauce, wasabi, and pickled ginger

Instructions:

1. Lay a nori seaweed sheet, shiny side down, on a spotless, level surface.

2. Evenly cover the nori sheet with a thin layer of cooked brown rice, leaving a 1-inch border around the top.

3. Along the bottom border of the rice, arrange the cucumber, avocado, carrot, red bell pepper, and tofu or crab sticks (if using) in a single line.

4. Roll the nori sheet firmly, starting from the bottom edge. You can form the roll with your hands or a bamboo sushi mat.

5. To seal the roll, dab the upper edge of the nori sheet with a little water.

6. Continue with the remaining fillings and nori sheets.

7. Cut each sushi roll into 6–8 pieces with a sharp knife.

8. Present the sushi rolls with dipping sauces of wasabi, pickled ginger, and soy sauce.

9. Savor right away.

4 servings

Prepare Duration: 20 minutes

Cooking time for brown rice is thirty minutes.

Nutritional Value (one roll, per serving):

- 200 calories

- 5g of protein

- 35g of carbohydrates

- 5g of fat

- 5g of fiber

These recipes are full of minerals and tastes, making them ideal for filling meals. Savor the nutritious and delectable food!

Four

Recipes for Dinner

✓ *Baked Cod with Herbs and Lemon*

Ingredients:

- Two filets of cod

- One finely sliced lemon

- Two chopped garlic cloves

- Two teaspoons olive oil

- One tablespoon finely chopped fresh parsley

- 1 tablespoon finely chopped fresh dill

- Season with salt and pepper

Instructions:

1. Turn the oven on to 375°F, or 190°C.

2. Transfer the fish fillets to a parchment paper-lined baking dish.

3. Drizzle the cod fillets with olive oil and season with salt, pepper, minced garlic, chopped parsley, and chopped dill.

4. Top each cod fillet with a slice of lemon.

5. Bake the fish for 15 to 20 minutes in a preheated oven, or until it is opaque and flakes readily with a fork.

6. Garnish with extra fresh herbs and lemon slices, if preferred, and serve hot.

Two servings

Cooking Time: 15 to 20 minutes

Nutritional Value: 250 calories per serving

25g of protein

- 3g of carbohydrates

- 15g of fat

- 1g of fiber

✓ *Stuffed bell peppers with Quinoa and Ground Turkey*

Ingredients:

- 1/2 cup cooked quinoa

- 1/2 pound ground turkey

- 1/2 cup diced onion

- 1/2 cup diced tomatoes

- 1/2 cup split and seeded bell peppers

- One tsp of Italian spice

- Taste and add salt and pepper as needed.

- Optional: 1/4 cup of shredded cheese

Instructions:

1. Preheat the oven to 375°F, or 190°C.

2. Brown the ground turkey in a pan over medium heat.

3. Fill the skillet with the chopped tomatoes, diced onion, cooked quinoa, tomato sauce, Italian seasoning, salt, and pepper. Simmer the vegetables for a further five minutes, or until they are soft.

4. Tightly put the turkey and quinoa mixture into each half of the bell pepper.

5. Transfer the filled peppers to a baking dish and secure with foil.

6. Bake the peppers for 25 to 30 minutes, or until they are soft, in a preheated oven.

7. During the final five minutes of baking, if preferred, top the stuffed peppers with shredded cheese.

8. Present warm.

Two servings

Cook for 35 to 40 minutes.

Nutritional Value:

- 300 calories per serving

25g of protein

- 25g of carbohydrates

- 10g of fat

- 5g of fiber

✓ *Tofu and Vegetable Skewers Grilled*

Ingredients:

- One slice of zucchini

- One cubed block of firm tofu

- One chopped yellow bell pepper

- One red onion, sliced into pieces

- One cup of cherry tomatoes

- Two teaspoons each of olive oil and balsamic vinegar

- Two minced garlic cloves

- One tsp of Italian spice

- To taste, add salt and pepper

- Soak wooden skewers in water for half an hour

Instructions:

1. Set the grill's temperature to medium.

2. Combine the olive oil, balsamic vinegar, salt, pepper, Italian seasoning, and minced garlic in a bowl.

3. Alternately thread the diced veggies and cubed tofu onto the wooden skewers.

4. Evenly coat the skewers by brushing them with the marinade mixture.

5. After preheating the grill, place the skewers on it and cook for 8 to 10 minutes, flipping them over occasionally, until the tofu is gently browned and the vegetables are soft.

6. Take the skewers from the barbecue and serve them hot.

Two servings

Cooking Time: 8 to 10 minutes

Nutritional Value: 280 calories per serving

- 18g of protein

- 20g of carbohydrates

- 15g of fat

- 6g of fiber

Ingredients:

- One big eggplant cut into circles

- A cup of breadcrumbs made with whole wheat

- Grated Parmesan cheese, half a cup

- Two beaten eggs

- Two cups sauce marinara

- One cup of mozzarella cheese, shredded

- Eight ounces of whole wheat pasta, prepared as directed on the package.

– New basil leaves as a finishing touch

Instructions:

1. Preheat the oven to 375°F, or 190°C.

2. Coat each eggplant slice with a mixture of grated Parmesan cheese and whole wheat bread crumbs after dipping it into the beaten eggs.

3. Transfer the oiled eggplant slices to a parchment paper-lined baking sheet.

4. Bake the eggplant for 20 to 25 minutes, or until it is soft and browned on top.

5. Cover the bottom of a baking dish with a coating of marinara sauce.

6. Place half of the slices of roasted eggplant over the marinara sauce.

7. Drizzle the eggplant slices with half of the shredded mozzarella cheese.

8. Continue by adding more layers of shredded mozzarella cheese, baked eggplant slices, and marinara sauce.

9. Bake for a further 20 to 25 minutes, or until the cheese is bubbling and melted.

10. Garnish with freshly chopped basil and serve hot over cooked whole wheat pasta.

4 servings

45 to 50 minutes for cooking

Value for nutrition (per serving, without pasta):

- 250 calories

- 12g of protein

- 15g of carbohydrates

- 15g of fat

- 5g of fiber

✓ *Chicken with Lemon Garlic and Roasted Vegetables*

Ingredients:

-   Two skinless, boneless chicken breasts

- Two teaspoons of olive oil

- Four minced garlic cloves

- One lemon, squeezed and sliced

- A teaspoon of thyme, dried

- Two cups of mixed veggies (carrots, broccoli, bell peppers, and zucchini)

- Garnish with fresh parsley

Instructions:

1. Set the oven's temperature to 400°F, or 200°C.

2. Combine the olive oil, salt, pepper, dried thyme, lemon zest, lemon juice, and chopped garlic in a small bowl.

3. Transfer the chicken breasts to a baking dish and cover them with the lemon-garlic marinade, making sure to turn them to coat all sides.

4. In the baking dish, arrange the mixed veggies around the chicken breasts.

5. Bake for 25 to 30 minutes, or until the chicken is thoroughly cooked and the vegetables are soft, in a preheated oven.

6. Take it out of the oven, then give it a few minutes to rest before serving.

7. Before serving, garnish with fresh parsley.

Two servings

Cook for 25 to 30 minutes.

Nutritional Value:

- 300 calories per serving

- 30g of protein

- 15g of carbohydrates

- 15g of fat

- 5g of fiber

✓ *Enchiladas with Sweet Potato and Black Beans*

Ingredients:

- 1 tablespoon olive oil

- 1 diced onion

- 2 minced garlic cloves

- 1 peeled and diced sweet potato

- 1 can (15 ounces) washed and drained black beans

- One teaspoon each of chili powder and ground cumin

- Eight whole wheat or corn tortillas

- Salt and pepper to taste

- 1 cup sauce for enchiladas

- One cup of shredded cheese, preferably Monterey Jack or cheddar; fresh cilantro for garnish

Instructions:

1. Turn the oven on to 375°F, or 190°C.

2. In a skillet over medium heat, warm the olive oil. Cook the minced garlic and diced onion until they are tender.

3. Cook the sweet potatoes in the skillet until they start to soften.

4. Add the chili powder, black beans, ground cumin, salt, and pepper. Simmer for an additional five minutes.

5. Use a skillet or microwave to reheat the tortillas until they are malleable and soft.

6. Top each tortilla with a dollop of enchilada sauce. Fill each tortilla with a spoonful of the sweet potato and black bean mixture. Roll each tortilla

up, tucking the seams under, and put in a baking dish.

7. Cover the rolled tortillas with the leftover enchilada sauce and top with shredded cheese.

8. Bake for 20 to 25 minutes, or until the cheese is bubbling and melted, in a preheated oven.

9. Before serving, garnish with fresh cilantro.

4 servings

30 minutes for cooking

Nutritional Value: 350 calories per serving

- 15g of protein

- 40g of carbohydrates

- 15g of fat

- 8g of fiber

✓ *Stir-fried Ginger Beef in Asian Style*

Ingredients:

- Thinly slice 1 pound of beef flank steak or sirloin

- Add 2 tablespoons of soy sauce

- One spoonful of sauce made from oysters

- One tablespoon of rice vinegar

- One tablespoon of brown sugar or honey

- Two minced garlic cloves

- 1 tablespoon finely chopped fresh ginger

- Cooked rice or noodles for dishing

- Two teaspoons vegetable oil

- Two cups mixed veggies (such as bell peppers, broccoli, and snap peas)

- Sesame seeds and fresh green onions for decoration.

Instructions:

1. Combine the soy sauce, oyster sauce, rice vinegar, honey or brown sugar, ginger and garlic powder, and minced garlic in a bowl. Let the steak sit in the marinade for 15 to 30 minutes after slicing it.

2. In a big skillet or wok, heat the vegetable oil over high heat. Stir-fry the marinated meat for two to three minutes, or until browned. Take out

and place aside the steak from the griddle.

3. Add the mixed vegetables to the same skillet and stir-fry for 3–4 minutes, or until they are crisp-tender.

4. Add the steak back to the skillet and mix it in with the veggies.

5. Top warm rice or noodles with the dish.

6. Before serving, garnish with sliced green onions and sesame seeds.

4 servings

15 minutes is the cooking time.

Value for nutrition (per serving; does not include rice or noodles):

- 300 calories

25g of protein

- 15g of carbohydrates

- 15g of fat

- 3g of fiber

Have fun!

Five

Snack Recipes

Ingredients:

- One can (15 ounces) of rinsed and drained chickpeas

- Two minced garlic cloves

- Two tablespoons lemon juice

- Two tablespoons tahini

- Two tsp olive oil

- Assorted fresh veggies for dipping (carrot sticks, cucumber slices, bell pepper strips)

- 1/2 teaspoon ground cumin

- Salt to taste

Instructions:

1. Put the chickpeas, olive oil, lemon juice, ground cumin, minced garlic, tahini, and salt in a food processor.

2. Blend until creamy and smooth, adding a little water as necessary to achieve the right consistency.

3. Taste and modify the seasoning to your liking.

4. Move the hummus to a serving bowl and, if like, top with a sprinkling of paprika and a drizzle of olive oil.

5. Present with a variety of fresh vegetable dips.

Servings: 4 Nutritional Value (assuming no vegetables):

- 150 calories

- 5g of protein

- 10g of carbohydrates

- 10g of fat

- 3g of fiber

✓ *Almond Butter on Apple Slices*

Ingredients:

- Two cored and sliced apples

- One-fourth cup almond butter

Instructions:

1. Use almond butter as a dip or spread it on apple slices.

2. Serve right away.

Servings: Two;   Each   Serving's
Nutritional Value:

- 200 calories

- 5g of protein

- 20g of carbohydrates

- 10g of fat

- 5g of fiber

✓ *Trail Mix including Dried Fruit and Nuts*

Ingredients:

- 1/2 cup of assorted nuts, including cashews, walnuts, and almonds

- 1/4 cup of dried fruit, like apricots, cranberries, or raisins

- Two teaspoons of chunky or chipped dark chocolate

Instructions:

1. In a bowl, combine dark chocolate chips, mixed nuts, and dried fruit.
2. Thoroughly stir to incorporate.
3. Divide into portion sizes and store in an airtight jar to use at a later time.

Servings: Two; Each Serving's Nutritional Value:

- 250 calories
- Six grams of protein
- 20g of carbohydrates
- 15g of fat
- 5g of fiber

✓ *Honey-topped Greek Yogurt with Walnuts*

Ingredients:

- One cup of Greek yogurt

- 1/4 cup chopped walnuts

- 2 teaspoons honey

Instructions:

1. Spoon Greek yogurt into a serving bowl.

2. Drizzle yogurt with honey.

3. Add chopped walnuts to the top.

4. Present right away.

Servings: 1

Calorie Value (per portion):

- 300 calories

20g of protein

- 25g of carbohydrates

- 15g of fat

- 2g of fiber

✓ *Pineapple Chunks with Cottage Cheese*

Ingredients:

- One half cup cottage cheese

- 1/2 cup chunky pineapple, either fresh or from a can

Instructions:

1. Spoon the cottage cheese into a bowl.

2. Add pineapple slices on top.

3. Present right away.

Servings: 1 Calorie Value (per portion):

- 150 calories

13g of protein

- 20g of carbohydrates

- Fat: 2 g

- 1g of fiber

✓ *Avocado with Whole Grain Crackers*

Ingredients:

– Six wholegrain crackers

- One mature avocado

- One tablespoon of lime juice

- One-fourth teaspoon each of salt and pepper

- Toppings that are optional: chopped cilantro, diced tomatoes, and red pepper flakes

Instructions:

1. In a bowl, mash the ripe avocado until smooth, adding lime juice, salt, and pepper.

2. Evenly distribute the guacamole over the whole grain crackers.

3. If desired, garnish with extra toppings.

4. Present right away.

Nutritional Value (per serving): 3 crackers with guacamole; 2 servings

- 150 calories

- 3g of protein

- 18g of carbohydrates

- 9g of fat

- 5g of fiber

✓ Rice Cake with Slices of Avocado and Tomato

Ingredients:

- One rice cake

- Half a sliced avocado

- A sliced tiny tomato

- Toppings: red pepper flakes, microgreens, salt and pepper to taste

Instructions:

1. Put the rice cake onto a dish.

2. Arrange tomato and avocado slices on top.

3. Add pepper and salt for seasoning.

4. If desired, garnish with extra toppings.

5. Present right away.

Servings: 1 Calorie Value (per portion):

- 150 calories

- 2g of protein

- 20g of carbohydrates

- 7g of fat

- 5g of fiber

These snack alternatives are filling and nourishing for any time of day because they include a good ratio of protein, healthy fats, and carbohydrates. Have fun!

Six

Dessert Recipes

Ingredients:

- One cup of mixed berries, including blueberries, raspberries, and strawberries

- One cup of Greek yogurt

- One tablespoon of maple syrup or honey

- 1/4 cup of granola

- Optional fresh mint leaves as a garnish

Instructions:

1. Clean the mixed berries and use a paper towel to pat dry. Slice and hull the strawberries, if using.

2. Thoroughly blend Greek yogurt with honey or maple syrup in a bowl.

3. Arrange granola, mixed berries, and Greek yogurt in serving bowls or glasses.

4. Continue layering until the bowls or glasses are full, and then top with a layer of mixed berries.

5. If preferred, garnish with fresh mint leaves.

6. When ready to serve, either serve right away or put in the fridge.

Two servings; ten minutes for preparation

Nutritional Value: 200 calories per serving

- 15g of protein

- 25g of carbohydrates

- 5g of fat

- 5g of fiber

✓ *Dark Chocolate-Coated Strawberries*

- 8–10 fresh strawberries, diced

- 4 ounces chopped dark chocolate

- 1 teaspoon optional coconut oil

Instructions:

1. Spread parchment paper over a baking sheet.

2. Heat the dark chocolate and coconut oil (if using) in 30-second increments in a microwave-safe bowl, stirring in between, until the chocolate is smooth and melted.

3. Using the stem as a support, dip each strawberry into the melted chocolate, swirling to ensure even coating.

4. Transfer the strawberries covered in chocolate to the baking sheet that has been ready.

5. Put the strawberries in the fridge for ten to fifteen minutes, or until the chocolate sets.

6. Present cold.

Two servings

15 minutes for preparation

Nutritional Value (for five strawberries per serving):

- 150 calories

- 2g of protein

- 20g of carbohydrates

- 9g of fat

- 4g of fiber

✓ Nutmeg and Cinnamon Baked Apples

Ingredients:

- 1 tablespoon melted butter or coconut oil

- 2 cored and halved apples

- 1 tablespoon honey or maple syrup

- 1 teaspoon ground cinnamon

- 1/4 teaspoon of nutmeg, ground

- Two teaspoons of optionally chopped pecans or walnuts

Instructions:

1. Turn the oven on to 375°F, or 190°C.

2. Combine the melted butter or coconut oil, honey, maple syrup, grated nutmeg, and cinnamon in a small bowl.

3. Arrange the apple halves, cut side up, in a baking dish.

4. Evenly coat the apple halves by brushing them with the cinnamon mixture.

5. Bake the apples for 20 to 25 minutes, or until they are soft, in a preheated oven.

6. Take out of the oven and top the baked apples with chopped pecans or walnuts, if using.

7. Present warm.

Two servings

Cooking Time: 20 to 25 minutes

Nutritional Value: 150 calories per serving

- 1g of protein

- 25g of carbohydrates

- 6g of fat

- 4g of fiber

✓ *Fresh Mint with Mango Sorbet*

Ingredients:

- 1/4 cup honey or maple syrup

- 2 ripe mangoes, chopped and peeled

– 1/4 cup of water

- New mint leaves for decoration

Instructions:

1. In a food processor or blender, combine water, honey (or maple syrup), and chopped mangoes.

2. Blend until creamy and smooth.

3. Transfer the mango mixture equally into a shallow dish by pouring it in.

4. Place plastic wrap over the dish and freeze for four to six hours, or until it solidifies.

5. Take the frozen mango combination out of the freezer and allow it to soften a little bit by letting it sit at room temperature for five to ten minutes.

6. Ladle the mango sorbet into glasses or serving bowls.

7. Add some mint leaves as a garnish.

8. Present right away.

4 servings

Ten minutes for preparation

Time to Freeze: 4-6 hours

Value of Nutrition (per serving):

- 100 calories

- 1g of protein

- 25g of carbohydrates

- Fat: 0 g

- 2g of fiber

Ingredients:

- Two ripe bananas, cut and peeled

- Two tablespoons almond butter

- One tablespoon maple syrup or honey

- One-fourth teaspoon vanilla extract

- Two tablespoons of chopped (optional) almonds

Instructions:

1. Arrange the sliced bananas in a single layer on a parchment paper-lined baking sheet.

2. Freeze the banana slices until they are fully frozen, which should take at least two hours.

3. After the bananas are frozen, put them in a blender or food processor.

4. Process the frozen banana slices in a blender until they are creamy and smooth, like ice cream.

5. In a small dish, thoroughly blend the almond butter, vanilla essence, and honey or maple syrup.

6. Pour the almond butter mixture over the ice cream with bananas.

7. If preferred, top with chopped almonds.

8. Serve right away.

Two servings

Ten minutes for preparation

Two hours is the freeze time.

Value of Nutrition (per serving):

- 220 calories

- 4g of protein

- 35g of carbohydrates

- 9g of fat

- 5g of fiber

✓ *Fruit-Garnished Greek Yogurt Popsicles*

Ingredients:

- One cup of Greek yogurt

- One tablespoon of maple syrup or honey

- A half cup of mixed fruit, including raspberries, blueberries, and strawberries

- Molds for popsicles

- Stick Pops

Instructions:

1. In a dish, thoroughly blend Greek yogurt with honey or maple syrup.

2. Clean and roughly chop the mixed fruit.

3. Using a spoon, add enough Greek yogurt to fill each popsicle, mold about one-third of the way up.

4. After the Greek yogurt layer, sprinkle a layer of mixed fruit on top.

5. Top over with a layer of Greek yogurt and continue layering until the popsicle molds are completely full.

Step 6: Place popsicle sticks inside the molds.

7. After the popsicles are fully frozen, place the popsicle molds in the freezer and freeze for at least 4 hours.

8. After the popsicles are frozen, run them under warm water for a brief period of time to extract them from the molds.

9. You can either serve it right away or freeze it in a zip-top bag.

4 servings

Ten minutes for preparation

Four hours is the freeze time.

Value of Nutrition (per serving):

- 70 calories

- 5g of protein

- 10g of carbohydrates

- Fat: 1 gram

- 1g of fiber

Ingredients:

- One-quarter cup chia seeds

- One cup of any kind of milk (almond, coconut, etc.)

- Two tablespoons cocoa powder

- One tablespoon of maple syrup or honey

- One-fourth teaspoon pure vanilla extract

- Fresh berries, optional as a garnish

Instructions:

1. In a bowl, thoroughly mix the chia seeds, milk, chocolate powder, vanilla essence, honey, or maple syrup.

2. To avoid clumps, let the mixture settle for five minutes before whisking it once more.

3. To let the chia seeds absorb the liquid and thicken, cover the bowl and place it in the refrigerator for at least two hours or overnight.

4. To guarantee a uniform consistency, stir the pudding just before serving.

5. Ladle the pudding with chocolate chia seeds into glasses or serving dishes.

6. If preferred, garnish with fresh berries.

7. Present cold.

Two servings; five minutes of preparation; two hours of chilling

Value of Nutrition (per serving):

- 150 calories

- 5g of protein

- 20g of carbohydrates

- 7g of fat

- 9g of fiber

These dessert dishes are the ideal way to indulge your sweet tooth without feeling guilty because they provide a delicious and healthier substitute for traditional candies. Have fun!

Seven

Beverages

✓ *Pineapple and Spinach Green Smoothie*

Ingredients:

- 1 cup sliced pineapple

- 1 cup fresh spinach leaves

- 1 ripe banana

- Half a cup of Greek yogurt

- Half a cup water or coconut water

- One tablespoon (optional) of maple syrup or honey

- Ice cubes, if desired

Instructions:

1. Put chopped pineapple, banana, Greek yogurt, fresh spinach leaves, and coconut water in a blender.

2. Blend until creamy and smooth.

3. If you want more sweetness, taste and add more honey or maple syrup.

4. If preferred, add the ice cubes and process until smooth once more.

5. Immediately serve after pouring into glasses.

Servings: Two; 5-minute prep

Nutritional Value: 150 calories per serving

- 5g of protein

- 30g of carbohydrates

- Fat: 1 gram

- 4g of fiber

✓ *Herbal Tea with Ginger and Lemon*

Ingredients:

- Two glasses of water

- Two tablespoons of loose herbal tea (such rooibos, peppermint, or chamomile)

- A cut 1-inch piece of fresh ginger

- One sliced lemon

- Taste-tested honey or maple syrup (optional)

Instructions:

1. Bring water to a boil in a small saucepan.

2. Turn off the heat and stir in the chopped ginger and loose herbal tea.

3. For five to ten minutes, cover and let soak.

4. Pour the tea through a strainer into cups and garnish with a lemon slice.

5. If preferred, sweeten with honey or maple syrup.

6. Enjoy the calming flavors while serving hot.

Two servings

Five minutes for preparation

Cooking Time: 5 to 10 minutes

✓ *Watermelon Cucumber Mint Cooler*

Ingredients:

- 1 lime juice

- 1/2 chopped and peeled English cucumber

- 2 cups cubed watermelon

- 1-2 cups cold water

- 1 tablespoon minced fresh mint leaves

- Cubes of ice

Instructions:

1. Put the diced cucumber, diced watermelon, lime juice, and fresh mint leaves in a blender.

2. Process until smooth.

3. Transfer the blend into a pitcher.

4. Stir thoroughly and add enough cold water to get the right consistency.

5. Place ice cubes in glasses, then top the ice with the watermelon cucumber mint cooler.

6. If preferred, garnish with extra mint leaves.

7. Serve right away and savor the revitalizing beverage.

Two servings; ten minutes for preparation

Nutritional Value: 60 calories per serving

- 1g of protein

- 15g of carbohydrates

- Fat: 0 g

- 2g of fiber

✓ *Flaxseed-Berry Blast Smoothie*

Ingredients:

- One cup of mixed berries, including blueberries, raspberries, and strawberries

- One mature banana

- Half a cup of Greek yogurt

- One spoonful of flaxseed meal

- 1/2 cup almond milk, or any other type of milk.

- Ice cubes, if desired

- Taste-tested honey or maple syrup (optional)

Instructions:

1. Put the mixed berries, banana, Greek yogurt, ground flaxseeds, and almond milk into a blender.

2. Blend until creamy and smooth.

3. If you want more sweetness, taste and add more honey or maple syrup.

4. If preferred, add the ice cubes and process until smooth once more.

5. Immediately serve after pouring into glasses.

Servings: Two; 5-minute prep

Nutritional Value: 150 calories per serving

- 5g of protein

- 25g of carbohydrates

- 3g of fat

- 6g of fiber

✓ *Lemon-infused Coconut Water*

Ingredients:

- One lime juice

- Two cups coconut water

- Ice cubes

- Optional lime slices as garnish

Instructions:

1. Pour the lime juice and coconut water into a pitcher.

2. Give it a good stir to combine.

3. Put ice cubes in glasses.

4. Cover the ice with the coconut water and lime combination.

5. Add a lime slice as a garnish to each drink.

6. Pour and enjoy the cool beverage right away.

Two servings

Five minutes for preparation

Nutritional Value (30 calories per serving)

- Protein: 0 grams

- 8g of carbohydrates

- Fat: 0 g

- Fiber: 0 g

✓ Turmeric-infused Golden Milk Latte

Ingredients:

- 2 cups milk (almond, coconut, or dairy milk work well)

- 1/2 teaspoon ground cinnamon

- 1 teaspoon ground turmeric

- One tablespoon of honey or maple syrup

- One-fourth teaspoon of powdered ginger

- One teaspoon of optional vanilla extract

- An optional pinch of ground black pepper

- For a garnish, grind some cinnamon.

Instructions:

1. Heat the milk in a small saucepan over medium heat, being careful not to boil.

2. Add the ground ginger, cinnamon, and turmeric, as well as honey, maple syrup, vanilla extract, and, if desired, a dash of crushed black pepper.

3. Keep whisking until the mixture is well cooked and the spices are well combined.

4. Fill mugs with the golden milk latte.

5. Sprinkle some ground cinnamon on top of each mug.

6. Pour hot and savor the delicious and cozy beverage.

Two servings

Five minutes for preparation

Five minutes to cook

Value of Nutrition (per serving):

- 100 calories

- 2g of protein

- 15g of carbohydrates

- 4g of fat

- 1g of fiber

✓ *Citrus Slices with Sparkling Water*

Ingredients:

- Two cups of sparkling water

- A variety of citrus pieces (grapefruit, orange, lime, and lemon, for example)

Cubes of ice

Instructions:

1. Put ice cubes in glasses.

2. Fill each glass with a variety of citrus segments.

3. Drizzle the ice cubes and citrus segments with sparkling water.

4. Gently blend by stirring.

5. Pour and enjoy the crisp, energizing beverage right away.

Two servings

Five minutes for preparation

Nutritional Value (0 calories, 0 grams of protein) per serving

- 0g of carbohydrates

- Fat: 0 g

- Fiber: 0 g

From the hydrating qualities of coconut water to the anti-inflammatory effects of turmeric in the golden milk latte, these drinks offer a variety of flavors and health advantages. Savor these delectable beverages!

Conclusion

In your pursuit of improved liver health, keep the following measures in mind as you proceed:

1. **Consult with Healthcare Professionals:** To keep an eye on your liver health and to answer any questions or concerns you may have, keep in frequent contact with your doctor, dietician, and other members of your healthcare team.

2. **Adhere to Dietary Guidelines:** Make sure you include the dietary guidelines described in this book into your everyday routine. A balanced diet high in whole grains, fruits,

vegetables, lean meats, and healthy fats should be your goal. Pay attention to portion sizes and steer clear of processed foods, added sugar, and bad fats.

3. **Remain Hydrated:** To promote hydration and liver function, consume an ample amount of liquids, including water, herbal teas, and hydrating drinks like coconut water.

4. **Remain Active:** Take regular breaks from physical exercise in accordance with your degree of fitness and health. Exercise supports weight

management, enhances circulation, and enhances general wellbeing.

5. **Exercise Self-Care:** Include stress-relieving activities in your daily routine, such yoga, meditation, or enjoyable hobbies. Make rest and sleep a priority in order to maintain the health of your liver and your general energy.

You can sustain the health of your liver and your general well-being by putting these strategies into practice and keeping a proactive attitude toward your well-being.

21 Day Meal Plan

Day 1

- Breakfast: Avocado Toast with Poached Eggs

- Lunch: Mixed greens with Grilled Chicken Salad

- Dinner: Baked Cod with Herbs and Lemon

- Snack: Veggie Sticks with Hummus

- Beverage: Herbal Tea with Ginger and Lemon

Day 2

- Breakfast: Almonds and Berries with Oatmeal

- Lunch: Lentil Soup with Tomatoes and Spinach

- Dinner: Stuffed bell peppers with Quinoa and Ground Turkey

- Snack: Almond Butter on Apple Slices

- Beverage: Watermelon Cucumber Mint Cooler

Day 3

- Breakfast: Omelet with spinach and mushrooms

- Lunch: Avocado and Turkey Wrap

- Dinner: Tofu and Vegetable Skewers Grilled

- Snack: Trail Mix including Dried Fruit and Nuts

- Beverage: Flaxseed-Berry Blast Smoothie

Day 4

- Breakfast: Parfait of Greek Yogurt with Granola and Honey

- Lunch: Black bean and Quinoa Salad

- Dinner: Whole Wheat Pasta with Eggplant Parmesan

- Snack: Honey-topped Greek Yogurt with Walnuts

- Beverage: Lemon-infused Coconut Water

Day 5

- Breakfast: Pancakes made of whole grains and fresh fruit

- Lunch: Lettuce Wraps with Tuna Salad

- Dinner: Chicken with Lemon Garlic and Roasted Vegetables

- Snack: Pineapple Chunks with Cottage Cheese

- Beverage: Turmeric-infused Golden Milk Latte

Day 6

- Breakfast: Fantastic Breakfast Bowl of Quinoa with Nuts and Seeds

- Lunch: Stir-fried Vegetables with Chickpeas

- Dinner: Enchiladas with Sweet Potato and Black Beans

- Snack: Avocado with Whole Grain Crackers

- Beverage: Citrus Slices with Sparkling Water

Day 7

- Breakfast: Cream cheese and smoked salmon bagel

- Lunch: Salad Nicoise with Salmon

- Dinner: Stir-fried Ginger Beef in Asian Style

- Snack: Rice Cake with Slices of Avocado and Tomato

- Beverage: Pineapple and Spinach Green Smoothie

Day 8

- Breakfast: Banana Walnut Smoothie

- Lunch: Grilled shrimp in a Greek salad

- Dinner: Stir-fried Ginger Beef in Asian Style

- Snack: Veggie Sticks with Hummus

- Beverage: Herbal Tea with Ginger and Lemon

Day 9

- Breakfast: Breakfast Burrito with Veggies

- Lunch: Sushi Rolls with Brown Rice and Vegetables

- Dinner: Baked Cod with Herbs and Lemon

- Snack: Almond Butter on Apple Slices

- Beverage: Watermelon Cucumber Mint Cooler

Day 10

- Breakfast: Mango-Chia Seed Pudding

- Lunch: Sweet Potato and Turkey Chili

- Dinner: Whole Wheat Pasta with Eggplant Parmesan

- Snack: Trail Mix including Dried Fruit and Nuts

- Beverage: Flaxseed-Berry Blast Smoothie

Day 11

- Breakfast: Avocado Toast with Poached Eggs

- Lunch: Mixed greens with Grilled Chicken Salad

- Dinner: Stuffed bell peppers with Quinoa and Ground Turkey

- Snack: Honey-topped Greek Yogurt with Walnuts

- Beverage: Lemon-infused Coconut Water

Day 12

- Breakfast: Almonds and Berries with Oatmeal

- Lunch: Lentil Soup with Tomatoes and Spinach

- Dinner: Tofu and Vegetable Skewers Grilled

- Snack: Pineapple Chunks with Cottage Cheese
- Beverage: Turmeric-infused Golden Milk Latte

Day 13

- Breakfast: Omelet with spinach and mushrooms
- Lunch: Avocado and Turkey Wrap
- Dinner: Chicken with Lemon Garlic and Roasted Vegetables
- Snack: Rice Cake with Slices of Avocado and Tomato
- Beverage: Citrus Slices with Sparkling Water

Day 14

- Breakfast: Parfait of Greek Yogurt with Granola and Honey

- Lunch: Black bean and Quinoa Salad

- Dinner: Enchiladas with Sweet Potato and Black Beans

- Snack: Avocado with Whole Grain Crackers

- Beverage: Pineapple and Spinach Green Smoothie

Day 15

- Breakfast: Pancakes made of whole grains and fresh fruit

- Lunch: Lettuce Wraps with Tuna Salad

- Dinner: Stir-fried Ginger Beef in Asian Style

- Snack: Veggie Sticks with Hummus

- Beverage: Herbal Tea with Ginger and Lemon

Day 16

- Breakfast: Fantastic Breakfast Bowl of Quinoa with Nuts and Seeds

- Lunch: Salad Nicoise with Salmon

- Dinner: Baked Cod with Herbs and Lemon

- Snack: Almond Butter on Apple Slices

- Beverage: Watermelon Cucumber Mint Cooler

Day 17

- Breakfast: Cream cheese and smoked salmon bagel
- Lunch: Stir-fried Vegetables with Chickpeas
- Dinner: Whole Wheat Pasta with Eggplant Parmesan
- Snack: Trail Mix including Dried Fruit and Nuts
- Beverage: Flaxseed-Berry Blast Smoothie

Day 18
- Breakfast: Banana Walnut Smoothie
- Lunch: Grilled shrimp in a Greek salad
- Dinner: Enchiladas with Sweet Potato and Black Beans

- Snack: Honey-topped Greek Yogurt with Walnuts

- Beverage: Lemon-infused Coconut Water

Day 19

- Breakfast: Breakfast Burrito with Veggies

- Lunch: Sushi Rolls with Brown Rice and Vegetables

- Dinner: Stuffed bell peppers with Quinoa and Ground Turkey

- Snack: Pineapple Chunks with Cottage Cheese

- Beverage: Turmeric-infused Golden Milk Latte

Day 20

- Breakfast: Mango-Chia Seed Pudding

- Lunch: Sweet Potato and Turkey Chili

- Dinner: Chicken with Lemon Garlic and Roasted Vegetables

- Snack: Rice Cake with Slices of Avocado and Tomato

- Beverage: Citrus Slices with Sparkling Water

Day 21

- Breakfast: Avocado Toast with Poached Eggs

- Lunch: Mixed greens with Grilled Chicken Salad

- Dinner: Tofu and Vegetable Skewers Grilled

- Snack: Avocado with Whole Grain Crackers

- Beverage: Pineapple and Spinach Green Smoothie

Enjoy your delicious and nutritious meals over the next 21 days!